Yoga for the Psoas

34 Stretches for the Deepest Core Muscle

Kalidasa Brown

ISBN-13:
978-1502874429

ISBN-10:
1502874423

First Printing, 2014

Printed in the United States of America

Yoga for the Psoas
34 Stretches for the Deepest Core Muscle

First Printing, 2014
Published in the United States of America

Liability Disclaimer

By reading this book, you assume all risks associated with using the advice given below, with a full understanding that you, solely, are responsible for anything that may occur as a result of putting this information into action in any way, and regardless of your interpretation of the advice.

You further agree that our company cannot be held responsible in any way for the success or failure of your business as a result of the information presented in this book. It is your responsibility to conduct your own due diligence regarding the safe and successful operation of your business if you intend to apply any of our information in any way to your business operations.

This book contains general information about medical conditions and treatments. The information is not advice, and should not be treated as such.

The medical information in this book is provided "as is" without any representations or warranties, express or implied. Kalidasa Brown makes no representations or warranties in relation to the medical information in this book.

Without prejudice to the generality of the foregoing paragraph, Kalidasa Brown does not warrant that: The medical information in this book will be constantly available or available at all; or the medical information in this book is complete, true, accurate, up-to-date, or non-misleading.

Terms of Use

You are given a non-transferable, "personal use" license to this book. You cannot distribute it or share it with other individuals.

Also, there are no resale rights or private label rights granted when purchasing this book. In other words, it's for your own personal use only.

Yoga for the Psoas

34 Stretches for the Deepest Core Muscle

Contents

Introduction

This yoga class contains 22 poses plus variations for a total of around 50 poses to stretch the psoas, the deepest muscle in the body. Only three poses are there for warmup, each with their own benefits. With all the variations you can easily create a stronger or easier class for yourself.

The class starts with a breathing exercise that will charge your body with life energy. That will help you to work deeper into the muscles for the best stretch.

This would be a very advanced class taking a couple of hours to complete if all the poses and variations were done. However, anyone can benefit from it by doing the easier versions of the poses.

You can also hold the poses for a shorter time to make it easier. Or, make it a much stronger class by lengthening the holding times as well as including the stronger variations of the poses.

While the poses are designed specifically for the psoas the whole body gets a workout because the psoas is central to so many movements. Only the head, neck, arms and lower leg movements don't involve the psoas being activated or pulled in some way.

The poses are described in detail with an accompanying photo so you can see and fully understand how to do each one as well as their variations.

While this yoga class can be for advanced students it is written so that people with little or no experience with yoga will be able to do the poses successfully.

At the beginning is useful information about the psoas. That is followed by an explanation of yoga and how to practice for full benefit and without injury or pain.

Each pose starts with a photo showing the main way to do the pose. Later photos show the variations as they are described.

About the Psoas

The psoas major muscle, or psoas for short, is the deepest muscle in the body. It runs from the upper inner thigh, the inside of the lesser trochanter, under all the other muscles and tissue toward the hip point in the front where it comes close to the surface of the body just to the inside of the prominent front hip bone, or the ASIS.

From there it continues through the lower torso toward the spine where it attaches to the inner lower back where it attaches to the forward part of the inner spine.

The number of places where it attaches to the vertebras in the lower back varies from person to person; usually from five to seven. This is the origin of the psoas muscle which is on the inner sides of the five lumbar vertebras. Sometimes the eleventh and/or twelfth thoracic vertebras also have attachments for the psoas.

A little less than half of all people also have a psoas minor. It is also stretched when the psoas major is stretched.

The purpose of the psoas is widely debated though most people agree that it's a hip flexor and external rotator. That is, it helps to lift the thigh and also to rotate the hip out.

A tight psoas can cause lower back pain by compressing the discs in the lower back. It can also pull the lower back forward which causes extra arch in the lower back which is called lordosis. Stretching the psoas can bring relief.

The psoas is very difficult to reach for massage or physical therapy. The only places that it can be accessed by tough is through the belly, just to the inside of the hip bone in front, and at the upper inner thigh attachment. There are also stretches that can have an effect on it, most of which are included in this book.

Doing Yoga
Poses Safely

When practicing yoga, or any exercise for that matter, there are ways you can practice that will insure that you have a good experience and get what you need and want out of your practice. The first concern, or course, is safety.

Safety is actually pretty easy. All you need to do is to avoid pain! Pain is your friend; it instantly tells you when something is not right for your body.

It doesn't matter what an instructor or anyone else says, your body is yours and it knows when something doesn't work for it. Its communication is simple and immediate: if it hurts, stop!

There is an old adage that says, "No pain, no gain." Well, I'm here to tell you that this is backwards. "Pain, no gain," is much more accurate. And, recent studies prove that this is the case in most exercise situations.

However, there are some kinds of pain that are good. Mainly the slight pain you get when you get a good stretch. Of course, there are limits to this as well.

The main thing is to avoid working the stretch to the point where you resist. Pushing through your body's natural resistance into a stretch is one of the best ways I know of to injure yourself.

Another great way to get a severe injury is to try to work through an injury. Reinjuring an injury, even a very minor one, can cost you a lot of time in healing.

A minor injury may take a week or two to heal, sometimes even less. Reinjuring that same injury can take six to twelve weeks or longer to heal.

Each body has its own limits. Knowing what your limits are is very important in staying safe with any exercise program.

To make maters more complicated, your body's limits can vary from day to day. In come cases they can even vary minute to minute. Avoiding pain is the best way to know what is ideal for your body at any given moment.

One of the best ways to work a stretch is to work up to the point of pain without actually going into pain. Holding a stretch for a long time is a good way to find just the right amount of pressure to put into a stretch. Take your time and you will find exactly what is right for you in each stretch you practice

Another thing to consider here is how long you have been practicing a particular stretch. If you are just starting out, or you find a muscle that you haven't really stretched for a long time, then you might consider a shorter holding time until you become familiar with that muscle. It is always a good idea to allow time for your body to get used to any new activity.

The main thing is to take your time and pay attention to what is happening in your body. This will prevent injury as well as give you the best stretch.

What Makes a Stretch Yoga

One of the differences between just stretching and doing yoga is the use of breath in your practice. Breathing into a stretch with focus on the affected muscle or muscles is one of the best ways for you to get the benefits of yoga. And, breath work in yoga practice can help prevent injury.

A strong focus on a stretch becomes a meditation that will increase the benefits. That focus doesn't have to be intense and unwavering. And, it doesn't take years to master. All you need to do is focus on the stretch as best you can. Your ability will increase over time.

Focus on feeling what is happening moment by moment. Stay present with your stretch and breathe as you stretch.

Your internal dialogue about what is happening will also affect your practice. It is amazing how deeply our own thoughts can influence the practice of yoga, usually in a negative way.

For example, you may have some judgment about a pose, about how well you think you are or aren't doing. Anything that gets in the way of you focusing on your practice is something that can be acknowledged internally and let go of.

In a class you might have other issues that may not come up when practicing alone. Comparing yourself to others or being competitive are two of the biggest issues that people sometimes have. Another is feeling awkward or self-conscious about how you look, especially when starting out.

Believe me, most people are not paying any attention to what or how you are doing at all. If they are, then that is an issue of theirs that they need to deal with!

The ideal place to be in with your yoga practice is to have no thoughts. This isn't something most people can do, but it is one of the things that yoga is designed to help the practitioner toward.

There is more to yoga that these guidelines, but that is a long discussion for another time. Feel free to let me know if you'd like to know more about something specific that I could add to future books.

The last thing I'll say about yoga here is to have fun with it. Yoga doesn't have to be a somber experience. In fact, it covers all aspects of the being.

In my classes I am pretty irreverent, making jokes and telling stories about yoga. I like to make my classes fun. You may not find that in my writings, but do bring some of your own fun into your practice.

Three Part Breath

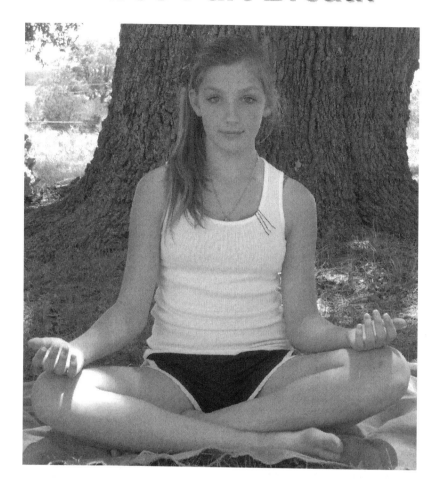

Starting with breathing exercises is good for centering, relaxing the body and for charging it with energy for the coming practice. One of the best breathing practices is a simple deep, full breath called the three part breath.

Start by sitting comfortably with your spine tall, preferably not leaning back against anything. This is important for the energy flow in the spine; however leaning is ok if your body is not comfortable without support.

Over time, as the body strengthens you will find it easier to sit without support. Sitting cross leg on the floor is ideal, but a chair can be more comfortable if you have a problem with sitting on the floor.

Sit with your hands and arms resting on your legs with the palms up. There is a tendency to press down if the palms are down. More importantly, the energy flows better when the palms are up.

This practice is called the three part breath because three areas of the lungs are filled from the bottom up. First, the belly is filled up to the diaphragm, then the lower chest is filled with air, and finally the breath continues to fill up into the upper chest.

At first it can be difficult to tell which area the breath is filling. Placing one hand on your belly and the other on your chest will let you know where the breath is going.

Inhaling through the nose and exhaling through the mouth is ideal because it is in alignment with how energy flows in the body.

Inhales and exhales should be slow and steady with a hold when the lungs are full. The length of the hold is whatever is comfortable for you. Ideally, the inhale, hold and exhale take about the same amount of time.

If you get out of breath you need to decrease the length of the hold or speed up the inhale and exhale time. You will get better at this over time.

Three Part Breath Short Instructions

Sit comfortably with your spine tall, hands on your legs palms up. Take a slow and steady inhale through your nose filling first the belly, then the lower chest and then the upper chest. Hold for a comfortable length of time and exhale slowly and steady through your mouth.

Neck Stretches

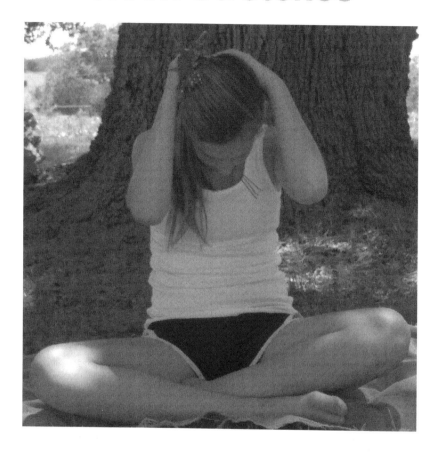

This set of poses and the next are warmups which help get the blood flowing in your body so it is ready for the stronger work to come. Warming up before any exercise is important to prevent injury and for maximum benefit.

The neck stretch is done while sitting with your body tall. Take a breath and exhale as you release your head down taking your chin toward the chest.

You can then use your fingertips on the back of your head to very gently help your head down and just a little forward.

Allow your upper back and shoulders to relax so that your elbows release down in front of you. Continue to relax your shoulders and arms as you gently allow the stretch to happen while you breathe into your neck muscles. Avoid pulling so hard that it hurts.

You can move the stretch to different areas of the neck by gently turning your head to the side. Work the stretch on that side, and then turn your head to work the neck on the other side. Try different positions to see what works best for you.

As you can see in the photo she's turned her head to her left. Be sure to stretch both sides like she's doing in the next photo. Work the stretch for a few breaths then release with an inhale to bring your head back up.

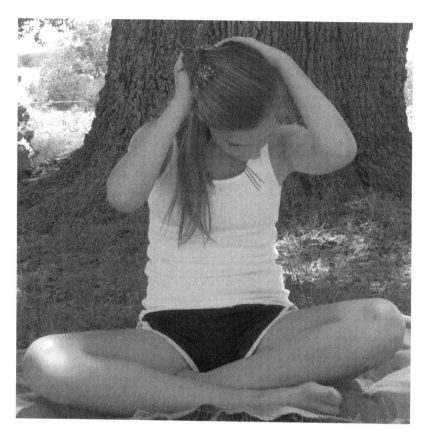

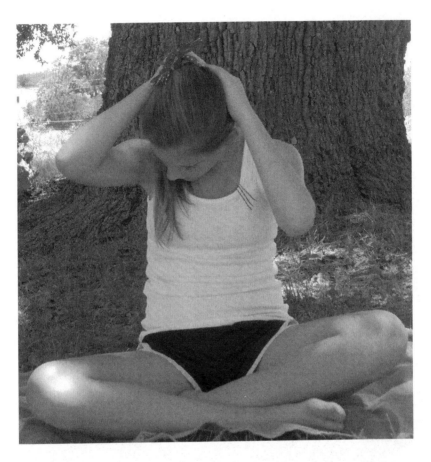

To stretch the left side of your neck, take another breath as you lengthen through your spine with your head extending up. As you exhale release your head to the right side.

Take your right hand over your head to the left side of your head and very gently draw your head to the right.

Extend your left arm off to the side with your hand a foot or so away from your body. Reach your left shoulder away from the neck so you feel a stretch throughout the whole arm.

You see her in the photo that she's flexing her hand back a little. You can flex it back as far as you need to bring the stretch into the hand.

Hold the extended arm for as long as is comfortable for you. She's continuing to hold the arm position as she does the other techniques but you can release your arm whenever you're ready, especially if it gets tired.

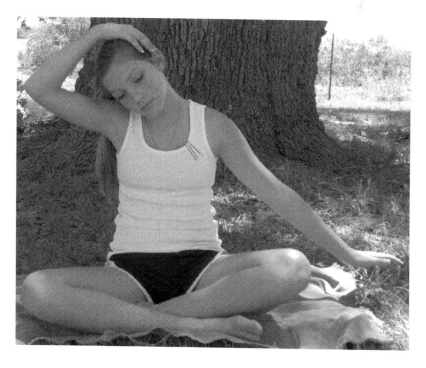

Once you've stretched the neck to the side for a few breaths you can move the stretch to different areas of the side neck by turning your head down or up. Be careful when you turn your head, pulling on the head while you're turning it can cause pain.

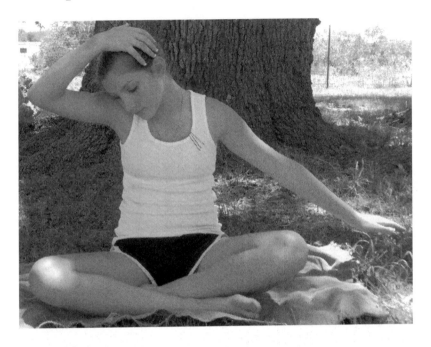

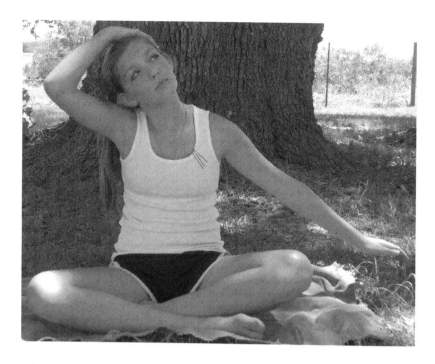

If you have any injury or any pain in the neck be very gentle and allow the stretch to happen slowly. Taking more time with these stretches will often relieve any neck pain.

Release with an inhale as you bring your head up, and then exhale as you let your head to the other side to repeat the techniques.

Shoulder Warm Up

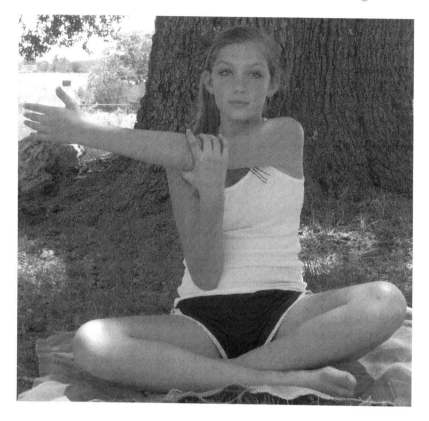

These shoulder warm ups are great for relieving tension in the upper back as well as the shoulders. There are many ways to move your arms to stretch different areas. Try different positions to find what is best for you.

Start sitting on the floor with a tall spine. Of course, you can use a chair if you like.

With an inhale, reach your left arm straight out in front of you. As you exhale, take it horizontally across your body in front of you. Use your right hand to help pull your arm in and to the right drawing the left shoulder to the right.

In the photo she's holding her arm. Some people like to reach all the way to the shoulder to draw it around. Try both to see what works best for you.

After you've worked the shoulder with your arm in this position for a few breaths, exhale as you let the arm drop down diagonally in front of you stretching your shoulder diagonally. Use your other arm to draw the arm in and more to the diagonal for the best shoulder stretch

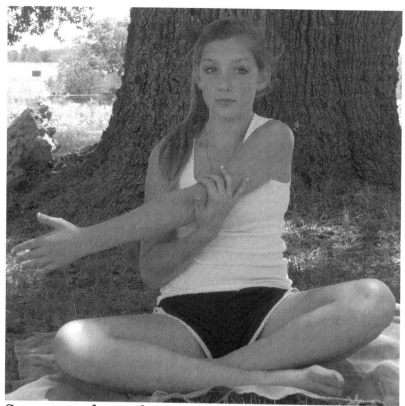

Some people prefer to use the right hand on top of the left arm rather than under. Whatever is comfortable for you is ideal.

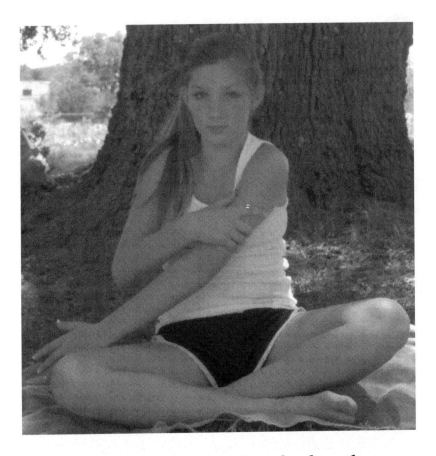

Work each of the stretches for a few breaths on each side. Ideally, you would take three or four minutes to do the whole shoulder series to thoroughly stretch your shoulders.

Bound Angle

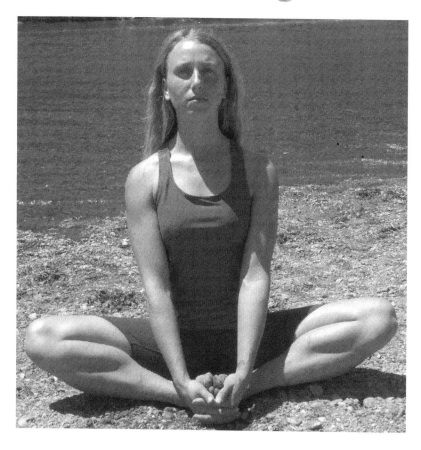

This stretch works the inner hip and groin area. It can also affect some of the muscles in the thigh. There is a hidden benefit to the upper back and shoulders when the shoulders are actively drawn down.

Start by sitting with the soles of your feet together. Interlace your fingers wrapping your hands around your feet.

Use your arm strength, the biceps, to pull your lower back in making the spine tall. Relax the shoulders so they drop down.

Actively reaching your shoulders down will give you a nice stretch in the upper back. Also, just pulling on your feet will help pull them down.

If that doesn't work for you, you can put your hands behind your back and press the floor to make your body tall. Turning your hands so your fingers are pointing back works best for most people, but adjust for what you like.

The closer your hands are to your hips, the taller your body will be. Do whichever technique is comfortable for you so that you get the best stretch possible.

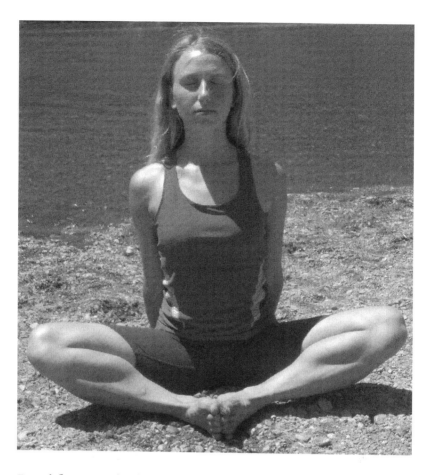

In either variation, use your leg strength to draw the knees down toward the floor to increase the stretch.

After you've warmed up for a few breaths you can use your hands, forearms, or elbows to gently press your knees down. These are strong muscles and can usually take a lot of pressure. Make sure you are fully warmed up in the area first though.

Or, wait till you've done the pose a few times before pressing very hard.

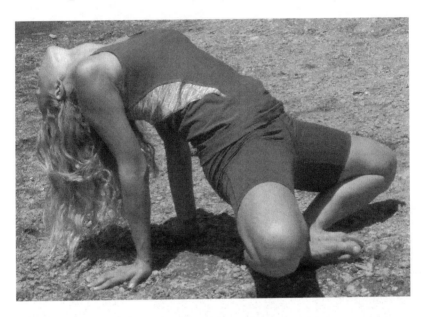

Once you have worked your knees down in bound angle for a few breaths it is time to move the stretch into the psoas. Place your hands a foot or so behind you so you can lean back.

Next, lift your hips and arch your back. Actively keep pressing your knees down as you press your hips forward and up.

She is fully arching her neck back nearly as far as she can. Be sure to arch just a little less than a full arch to protect the discs from compression.

There is a type of activation in the lower back that helps increase the psoas stretch in all back arching poses. That is to slightly flatten the lower back once you're in the pose.

The movement is often very slight. Sometimes there isn't even any movement at all. Sometimes just the activation of the muscles to flatten the lower back is all that is needed to increase the psoas stretch.

It may take time to develop the ability to do that subtle movement or activation. It will get easier with practice. And, it is mentioned in all the back arch poses, so you'll have plenty of opportunity to practice it.

Camel Pose

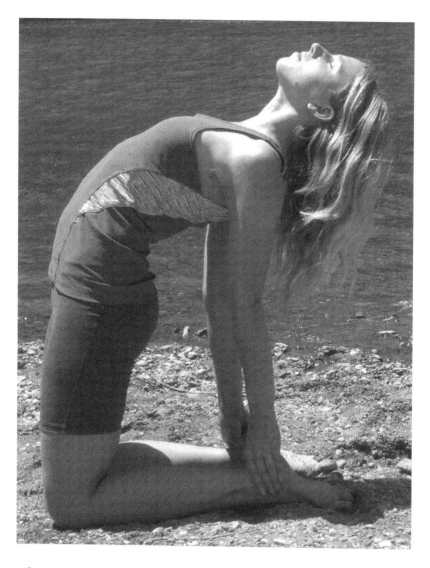

The psoas will stretch pretty much any time you do a back arch. Camel is one of the best back arches because there are many modifications that can make the pose either very easy, or very strong. We'll start with the easier techniques first.

For most people, the easiest Camel Pose is done with the hands on the hips. This is also a good way to warm up your back for future back bending. And, you can get a great stretch with this simplified version.

One caution for doing any back bending pose is to avoid overarching your neck. In all but the last version of Camel she is not arching her neck much at all. You can arch yours further if you like, but avoid arching as far as it will go.

You can also arch less if needed. Simply keep your chin to your chest while doing the pose. Just take care of your neck!

Overarching your neck causes a compression to the discs in the neck. The individual vertebras move toward each other on the back side causing them to press on the disc in between.

This can cause injury by gradually eroding the disc. It can also aggravate an existing injury which can cause an even greater injury.

That can be eliminated by lifting your head just an inch or two from a full arch. That will usually prevent these types of injuries.

Or, reduce the arch even more by only arching your neck a little. Keeping your chin to the chest will keep your neck completely safe.

The beginning position for Camel pose is kneeling upright. Use a pad under your knees as needed for comfort.

Place your hands on your hips and lower back. Come into the pose by inhaling tall, and arching your back as you continue filling your lungs. Arch into a comfortable position with your arms supporting the weight of your upper body on your hips.

Hold the pose for a few breaths. Inhale to come up out of the pose.

If your back is not strong enough to come out by lifting, or if there is pain, then you can sit down out of the pose. Simply exhale as you release to sitting on your heels.

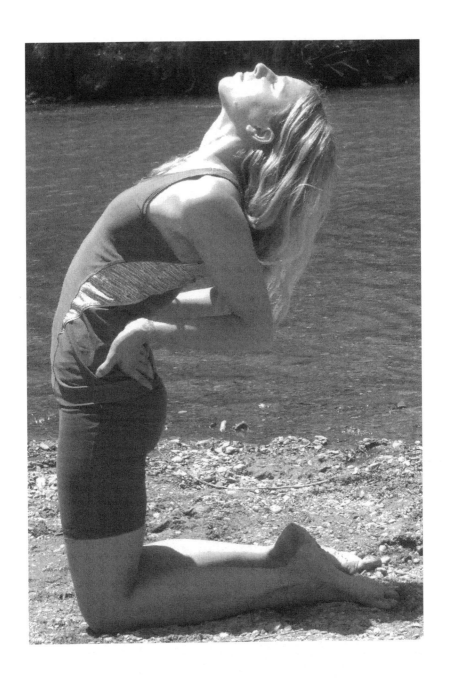

A deeper Camel is done by placing your hands on your feet for support. Start by sitting on your feet with your toes turned under on the floor and your hands on your heels.

With an exhale, press your hips up and away from your feet. Support your upper body's weight with your hands on your heels. Press your hips away to fully activate the pose.

Alternately, you can come into the pose from a kneeling position. This is the usual way it is taught, but I present it second because it can strain your back if you are new to the pose, don't have a deep back arch, or if you lack strength. It is best to practice Camel by pressing up into it from sitting before trying this one.

From kneeling with your feet up on the toes, reach your hands back and down to your heels as you inhale. Avoid twisting to reach one hand down at a time because twisting as you arch can cause the back to go out of alignment. It can also cause other problems, especially if there is an existing back weakness.

Come out of the pose with in inhale as you bring your body up. Or, you can sit down on your heels to avoid straining your back.

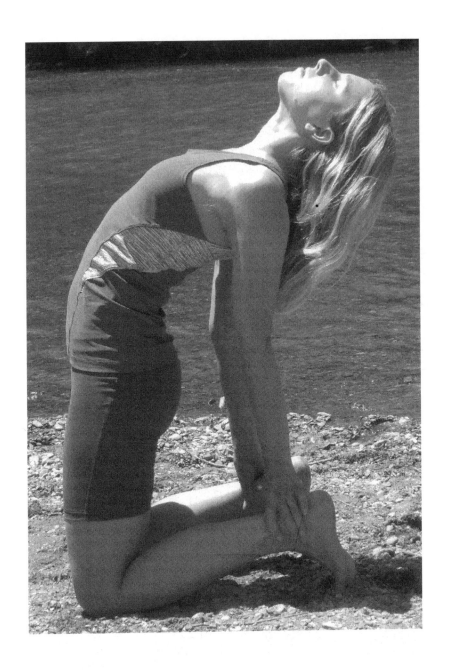

The strongest variation, the one shown in the first photo, is done the same way as the previous version. The only difference is to do the pose with the tops of your feet on the floor. This version gives the deepest back arch.

You can make either of these variations easier by using blocks on either side of your feet to rest your hands on. You work the by pressing your thighs away from you once you are set up and comfortable in the pose.

The final variation works into the psoas one side at a time. For some people it can be a better psoas stretch than the full Camel Pose.

Start by sitting on your right foot with the left on the floor in front of you. Press your left foot into the floor to lift your hips into the pose. The psoas on the right side will get the stretch. Be sure to work both sides.

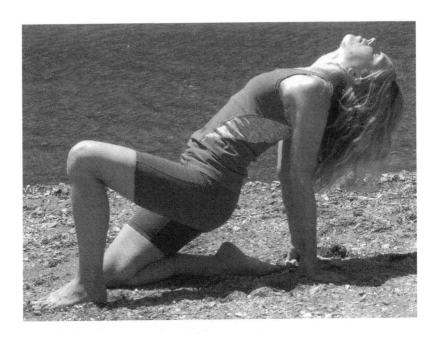

In all variations you can increase the psoas stretch by slightly flattening the lower back. This is hard to do since this is a back arch, but even a little activation in that direction will help.

That slight movement will also make the stretch safer for your back by decreasing the compression on the discs in the back. That compression is there in any back arch pose, so it is best to work on decreasing the arch whenever doing a back arch type pose, especially if you do a lot of back arch poses.

Lunge

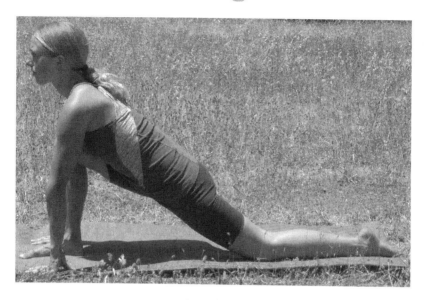

This is a great general stretch that stretches many muscles in the hips and legs. Several other areas of the body are also stretched and worked with the many variations that are possible with Lunge.

Start with your left knee down behind you and your right foot in front of you with your knee over the ankle. Use your hands on the floor or blocks for support.

Use a pad under your back knee for comfort if you need. Yoga is about being or getting comfortable, so do whatever it takes to feel great in all poses.

It is important to get the maximum stretch in the back leg that you can. You may need to hold the pose for a few breaths until the muscles loosen enough for you to move that back leg as far back as you comfortably can for the best stretch for you.

Be sure to keep your right knee above the right ankle, or at least no further forward than the toes. This alignment is important for knee safety.

Next, allow your hips to relax downward. There is a great release that often happens in the lower hip and groin area. This can also be a very strong stretch, so pay attention to that area as your hips move down. Move slowly here, especially if you aren't used to doing Lunge Pose.

Once you feel that you have found the best stance for your Lunge Pose, you can increase the stretch significantly in the front part of your back thigh. You do this by slowly bending your right knee forward.

Do this slowly because the extra stretch can happen very quickly. Pay attention to the front of your back thigh as well as your lower hip area when you make that shift.

Be careful not to let your front knee go further forward than your toes with that shift. Instead, increase the length of your stance if you need. You may find yourself needing to change your stance often as the muscles loosen up.

The psoas will stretch in this version of Lunge Pose, especially if it is tight. Other variations to come will increase that stretch significantly.

First, try the active Lunge. It doesn't generally stretch the psoas, but is a great pose for increasing strength, stretching the calf and Achilles tendon, and for how it can help with lower back pain.

Start in the Lunge you just did. Turn your back toes under, take a breath and with the exhale press your back leg straight as strongly as you can. Press the back heel away and keep actively pressing it away to stretch the calf and Achilles tendon.

Pressing that back heel away is often confusing to the brain simply because it isn't a movement that is usually done. You can help your brain create new neuro pathways by bringing that heel forward, then pressing it away from you.

This works because the brain can learn from the opposite. Usually it only takes one to three repetitions of this movement for the brain to remember how to move that way for the rest of your life.

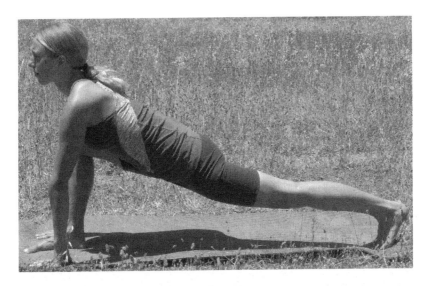

After you've held either of the above versions of Lunge for a few breaths it's time to start activating the psoas stretch. The first step is to come into Supported Lunge.

Starting from Lunge, lift your upper body so you're supporting yourself with your hands on your front knee or thigh.

Ideally, this will create an arch in your lower back. The psoas on the left side should get a stretch in this position, as long as you have a good distance between your front foot and back knee. Increase that stretch with the subtle movement of slightly flattening your lower back.

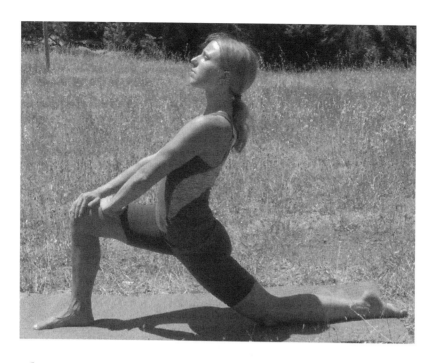

The next pose to try is a variation of Warrior One. Warrior One is included later, and this version is a good alternate as well as a great warm up for Warrior One.

The main benefit to this pose is that it increases the back arch and therefore the psoas stretch. The arms reaching overhead help lengthen the torso which will help to slightly flatten the lower back arch.

From supported Lunge reach your arms overhead. Reach strongly upward through your arms and torso to fill out the back arch which will help to slightly draw your lower back out. .

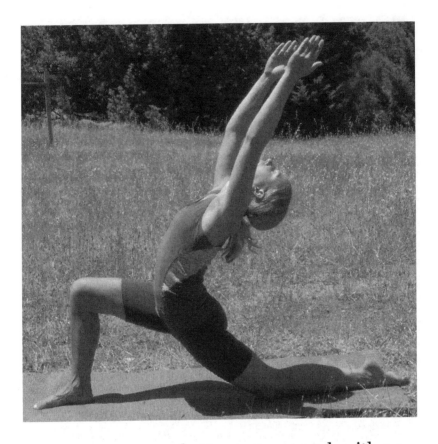

You can get an ever better psoas stretch with a Side Bend Lunge. The psoas runs through the torso, so bending to the side away from it draws it even longer giving it a nice stretch.

From Supported Lunge, inhale your left arm up alongside your head, and then exhale over to the right. Continue to support your body with your right hand on your leg or hip. The deeper you can bend to the right side the stronger the stretch will be in the left psoas.

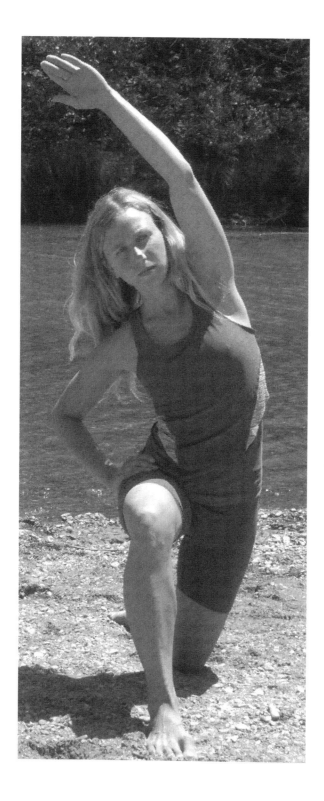

The next variation can also be a very strong psoas stretch. It is also one of the best stretches there is for stretching the muscles in the front of the thigh.

Start in Supported Lunge. You may need to shorten the distance between your legs for balance.

A shorter stance can lessen the psoas stretch somewhat, so keep the stance as long as possible. Do the pose next to a wall or chair if you need balance help.

Then, reach back with your left hand and draw your left foot forward toward your left hip. The quadriceps, or front of the thigh, will stretch with this move. This can be very strong stretch that comes on very quickly. So, go slowly and be careful not to overdo it.

The psoas stretch can also be increased here by arching your back as best you can. Slightly flattening your lower back will also help. Even a slight activation in that direction can help a lot.

From here, try shifting your front knee slightly forward. Move slowly because this is a strong adjustment for this pose. Only a slight modification is needed to affect big changes through all areas this pose stretches.

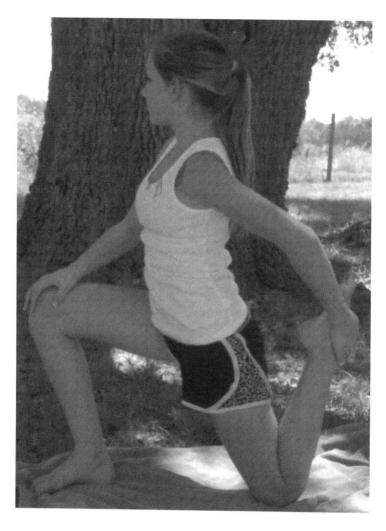

You can do the same pose with your back foot up a wall. This modification is helpful because you can focus on the subtle adjustment in the pose rather than focusing on holding your back leg, or dealing with your balance.

Focus on arching your back along with that slight flattening of the lower back. Use your hands on your knee or thigh to strongly press yourself as deep into the arch as you comfortably can.

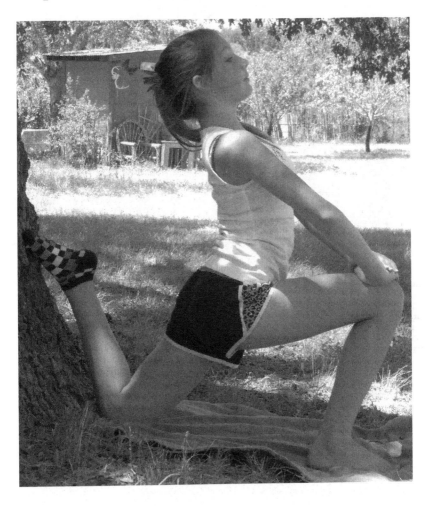

Psoas Reclining Stretch

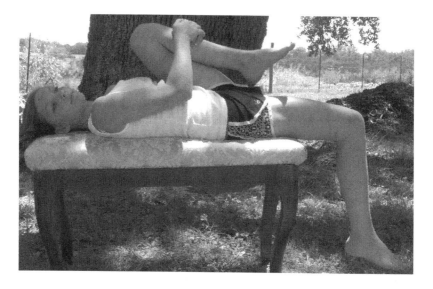

The variations that are possible for this pose help to make it work really well for most people. Having a friend help can give you one of the best posas stretches possible.

Start by lying down comfortably on a table or bed with your legs hanging off the end. Ideally you would be on something high enough so that your feet don't reach the floor but are close to it. Check the photo above to see what position you are ultimately looking for.

Hug your left knee into your chest. This is a great stretch for the lower back. It will also stretch the right psoas if it is fairly tight.

In the photo you see she has her hands across the front of the shin. If you have any kind of knee issue, if there's a pain in the knee or any tightness, then it will benefit you to hold on back of the thigh instead so that you are not compressing your knee. In other words, have your hands under your calf holding your thigh.

As you hug your knee in toward your chest, also draw it slightly up toward your head. This is a great all around stretch for the lower back, hip and leg. It is also a good warm up for the next part of the stretch.

Release the left leg and place the sole of that foot on the surface you're lying on. Shift over so your right leg drops down to the side. See what the stretch feels like for you with the right leg being lower than before.

Each part of this sequence can work the psoas with the stretch increasing with each position. Be sure to go slow to make sure you are not over doing it.

Next, draw your right foot back and place the top of the foot on the floor. See what that feels like.

The strongest stretch comes as you start to move your right foot back toward your head. This is a very strong stretch, so take this part especially slow. You can use a strap or towel around the foot to help draw it back.

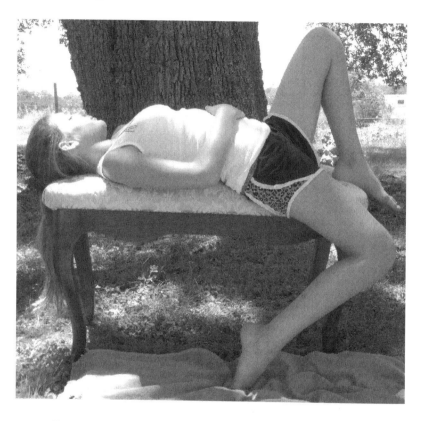

Another excellent way to do this stretch is to have a friend help pull your leg back. Guide them to do this slowly because this is a very strong stretch.

As they draw your foot back, have them also guide your thigh in the direction it is pointing; away from your hip, and with just a little pressure on your thigh. That movement is subtle, but strong. The strongest stretch comes from the knee moving down.

Psoas Couch Stretch

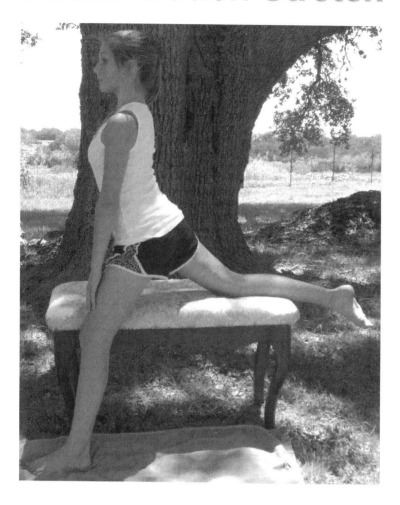

This stretch needs to be done with the back leg on a table or couch, something a little higher than a bed for most people. Use whatever works well for your height.

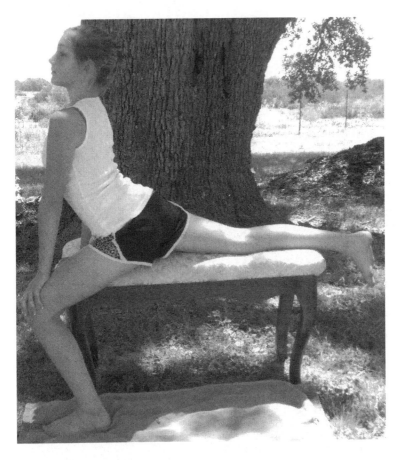

Take your right leg back as far as you can on the surface you're using while standing on your left leg. The standing leg can be in front of the surface or beside it like she's doing in the photo.

Adjust your position according to how you fit on the surface you are using. Notice how her right leg is a little further back in the second photo than in the first. She didn't move the leg back, rather her hips went slightly forward as she went down.

Keep your torso tall by using your hands on the front thigh to press you up. You might be able to press on the surface you're using. However, if you lift too far the back leg may raise in such a way as to decrease the stretch.

Try arching back slightly for even more stretch. Be sure to activate your lower back toward slightly flattening it for the best psoas activation.

Warrior Two

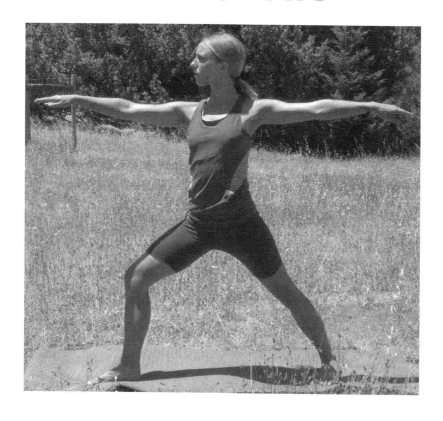

The next few poses are great for stretching the upper legs as well as the psoas. They can also build your leg strength, especially if you hold the poses for a longer time.

Start with your feet wide, right toe to the right, left foot turned in sharply. Ideally, you want your left toe to line up and point in the same direction as the left knee. This knee and toe alignment is mainly important to keep the knee from being injured.

The ideal starting position is a fairly wide stance. However, some people will need to take a narrower stance, especially when first starting out. If that is the case, gradually widen your stance as you get better at doing these poses.

As you inhale, bring your arms up to horizontal. Exhale bending your right knee to right over the ankle.

Widen the stance if you want to go deeper. Keep your front knee over the ankle to keep stress off your knee. If your knee goes past being over the toe you could injure your knee.

For safety your front knee needs to be right over the ankle in both directions that it can move; front to back as well as side to side. The activation that really brings in the stretch to the psoas is moving that knee back.

The deepest you would want to go into Warrior Two is with that right thigh parallel to the floor while maintaining the knee over the ankle. This is a very deep and strong position that is not necessary for a good psoas stretch.

Once you're here, you want to focus for a moment working with your stance to get it nice and solid. Make sure your feet are planted well and you're comfortable in the pose with your body being well balanced and grounded.

Activate your back leg by strengthening the leg so the thigh rotates back. This is called an outer rotation.

One way to help clarify the outer rotation is to think about pointing your knee more back behind you rather than having it pointing forward. It obviously won't move far, but in that direction.

Drawing your front knee back is fairly easy. It can easily move too far back taking it out of alignment. The active back leg (rotating back) will pull the front knee forward keeping it in proper alignment.

Doing this causes the two legs to pull in opposite directions. This creates a great stretch in the front hip and groin area. You can think of this action as being like a scissor opening. These actions are what really stretch the psoas, mostly in the front leg.

Keep your body tall in this pose. Lift from the top of the sternum to help draw your spine long and tall.

With a strong torso lift the lower back will likely start to arch. Draw your belly in to counter this arch. This will slightly flatten the lower back for an even greater psoas stretch. This is a pelvic tilt which is important for stretching the psoas.

The deeper Warrior Two is shown below. She isn't as deep as possible with the thigh parallel to the ground, but the psoas stretch will be a little better than in the first photo.

The first photo is a good stance for beginners. The distance between her feet is good while not too strong for most people. The second photo below is the perfect stance for her height.

Notice how relaxed and dropped her shoulders are in the pose. You can hardly tell that she is actively reaching her arms away from each other. The stretch in the upper back can be phenomenal when the arms are actively reaching away from each other.

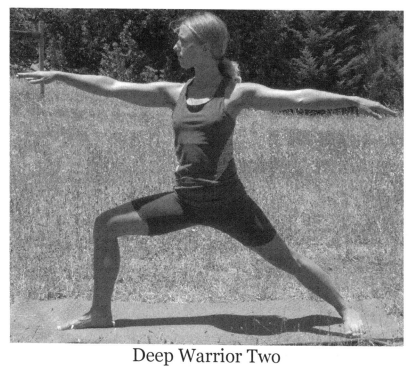

Deep Warrior Two

Modified Warrior Two

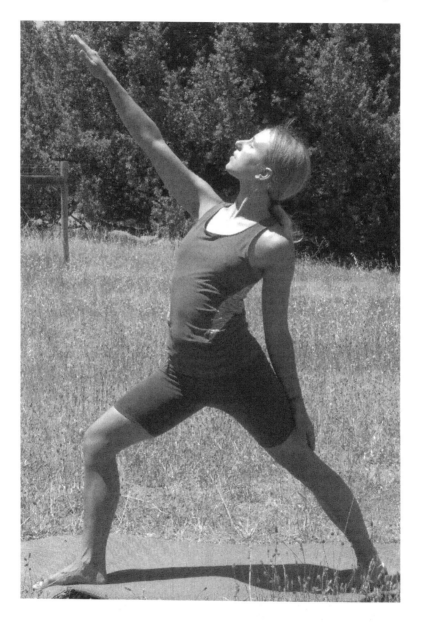

The posas stretch from Warrior Two is increased when doing this modification due to the back bend.

From warrior two take your back hand down and place it on your back leg. Your right arm reaches up in a diagonal direction. Reach both arms away from each other to maximize the upper back stretch.

Avoid leaning on your back leg with your left hand. Instead, allow it to rest on the leg with no more than the weight of your arm.

Reaching strongly through your right arm will help draw your lower back slightly flatter. Keep arching and reaching for a nice increase in the lower back stretch as well as the psoas.

Warrior One

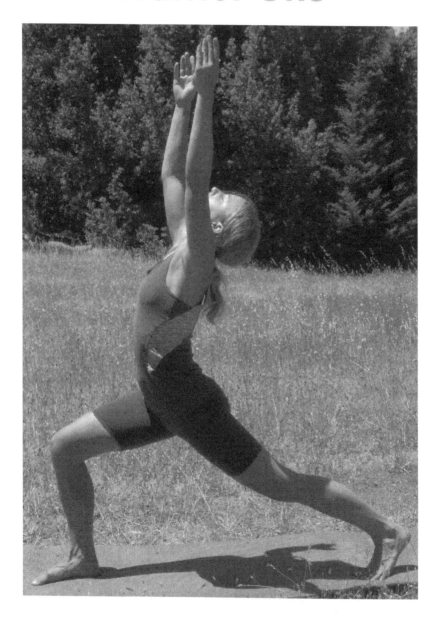

This pose is similar to the Arching Lunge presented earlier. It is a stronger pose, harder to do, but when done right the psoas will get more of a stretch than the Lunge version.

Start by coming into Warrior Two as above. Take another breath and exhale as you rotate your body to the right so you're facing over your right leg.

Also, rotate your hips to the left as you turn squaring them up over the front leg. Also, allow your back foot to roll up on the toe as that leg is drawn around.

Take your arms overhead as you rotate. Keep your arms parallel as you reach strongly through the arms and torso. Reach through the shoulders as well.

Once you're in position, press your left heel back toward the floor. If you are very flexible your heel may reach the floor though the foot won't be straight, rather it will roll down and be at a sharp angle.

Keep your back leg activated so you are pressing the outer edge of the foot into the floor. With sufficient activation the arch of the foot will lift.

It is common to have trouble knowing which way is back when pressing the heel back. You can teach your brain which way back is by taking your heel forward, then back again.

Look up between your arms so your neck is arched. Avoid overarching by reaching your head up lengthening through your neck to open up the arch.

The psoas stretch comes from several actions. Keeping the front knee actively working back countered by the strong back leg as done in Warrior Two is one.

Another is the left hip trying to rotate back with the strong back leg. Keep drawing it forward so your hips stay squared up over the front leg.

The last activation for the psoas is the combination of the lower back arch and the long reach through your arms that will draw that area more flat.

With all that going on, Warrior One is a very active pose that works or stretches almost the entire body. This is one of my favorite poses when done right!

Side Angle Stretch

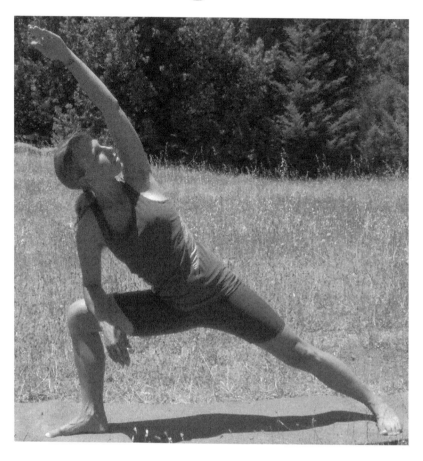

This pose is really great for the psoas both because of the position, which is similar to Warrior Two, and because you can assist in working the knee back with your arm.

Come into Warrior Two as above. With your next exhale, reach out long to the right and place your right forearm on your right thigh. At the same time take your left arm up alongside your head.

Rotate your torso and head so that you are looking up under your left arm toward the ceiling. Continuously rotate your torso strongly up throughout the pose.

Rotating your chest toward the ceiling will cause your right knee to pull forward and out of alignment with the ankle. Counter this by pressing your knee back with your forearm which will also help you rotate your torso up.

Reach long through your upper side; the arm reaches diagonally while your back leg is strongly rotating back as it is pressed away. The stretch through the upper side is one of the great benefits of this pose.

Keep your lower back long and slightly flattened for the best psoas stretch. The long reach through the upper side will help to tuck your pelvis.

Tree Pose

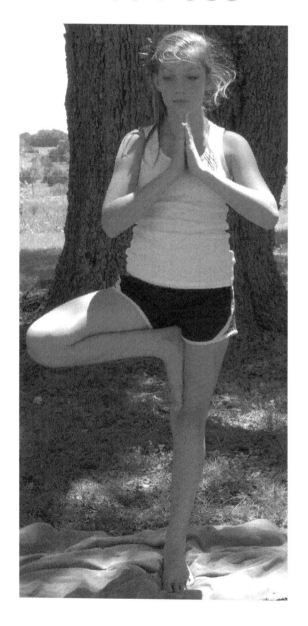

Start by standing with your feet parallel and about hip width apart. Shift your weight forward and back slightly to find balance between the heels and balls of your feet. Then, slightly shift side to side to balance your weight between the feet.

This simple standing position is actually a balance pose even though you are standing on both feet. Continue shifting your weight until you find a comfortable and solid balance before proceeding.

Once you're balanced, drop your weight into your left foot. Raise your right foot and place it high up on the left inner thigh. You can use your hand to help bring the foot up.

Balance can be an issue for some people. If that's the case, stand next to a wall with it on your left side, or have a chair that you can hold on to with your left hand.

It's good to hold on because if you're struggling with the balance you can't work the muscles, which means you won't get a good psoas stretch. It's better to let go of the balance part of the pose to get the stretch, at least for part of the pose.

A good practice to improve balance is to switch back and forth from holding on for balance and letting go when you are feeling balanced again.

Working with your balance like that will help improve your balance both in the poses and in general. It doesn't take long for some people to notice that they feel more balanced when simply walking.

Staring at a point in front of you is another way to help your balance in any balance pose. Staring at a point on the floor in front of you also works.

Grounding is another way to help with balance. To ground, start with feeling your feet before coming into the pose. Feel how they are solid in the floor. Then, let your energy drop down into the earth. Grounding takes practice, but it can have an amazing effect with even a little attention.

Once you are solid in the Tree Pose bring your hands into a prayer position in front of your chest. Take a few breaths in the pose as you work the stretch.

You work the stretch into the psoas by keeping your spine tall while tucking your pelvis to slightly flattening the lower back. Using your leg strength, draw your right knee back. Avoid letting your hips to turn back as well; keep them facing forward.

Drawing your upraised knee back while keeping your hips squared up forward is what stretches the psoas. The pelvic tilt slightly flattens the lower back and increases the stretch.

Lengthening through the spin tends to make the lower back arch. Continue working the pelvic tilt as you lengthen through your entire spine.

The hand position is not important for the psoas stretch, so holding on to something for balance is fine. But, if your balance is good, you can get some great stretches in your upper chest, upper back and shoulders by working with the hand position.

First, take your hands an inch or two overhead with your palms pressing together. With your palms actively pressing together draw your elbows back. This will stretch your chest and shoulders.

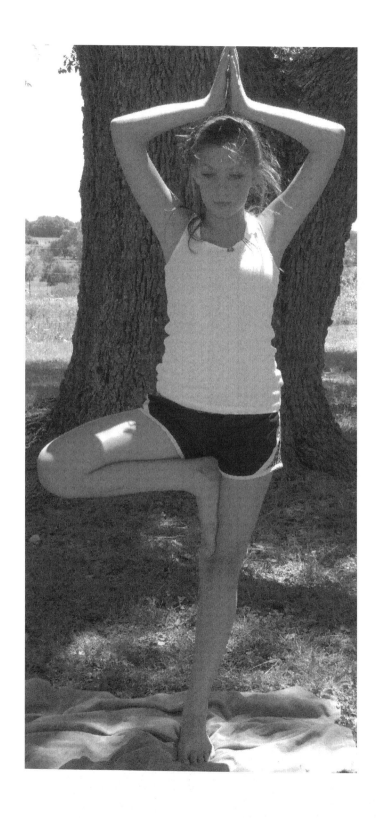

You can really increase that stretch to the chest by taking your hands behind your head with your fingers pointing down behind you. Work the stretch for a few breaths in this position.

Then, take another breath and with the exhale reach your hands overhead to a parallel position.

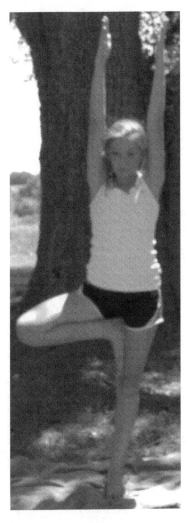

Keep reaching your hands up as well as activating your up raised knee back as you take a few breaths in the pose.

In the photos she has her foot in the ideal location very high up on the thigh. Lower is fine, the psoas will still be stretched.

A caution here is to avoid pressing your foot against the side of the knee if at all possible because you can hurt your knee that way.

Another possibility is to use a strap or towel to hold your foot up. You can still get a good psoas stretch by activating the knee back while holding it up with a prop.

Dancers Pose

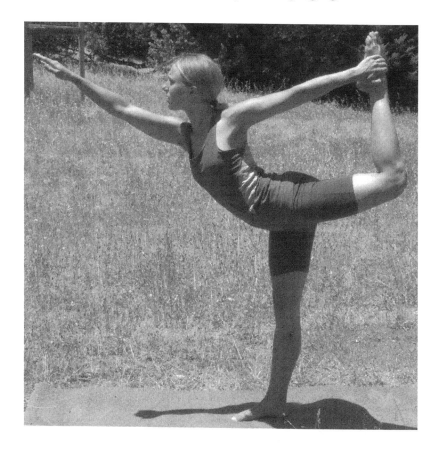

This is another balance pose that you can use a wall or chair to help with. Start by facing the wall or chair. You can try the pose out quickly just to find the right range before coming into it properly.

Instead of using a wall you can reach your hand through a doorway so you have something to hold on to without it being in the way. Once in the pose remember to let go from time to time to work with your balance.

Start with your feet parallel about hip width apart. Shift your weight side to side and front to back to equalize your weight between your feet and with about equal weight between the heels and balls of your feet.

Once you are solid and balanced drop your weight into your right foot and take hold of your left foot from behind with your left hand. Draw your back leg up behind you. Reach your right hand out in front.

You can use a strap or towel around the back foot if you can't reach it comfortably.

Use your arm strength to pull the back leg up. The arch and working that leg up are what gives the psoas stretch.

Press your back leg away as you hold on with your hand. Reach the opposite arm in front to create a counter pull. The muscles pulling against each other like this will increase your back arch and the psoas stretch. Breathe in the pose as you focus on the stretches that you feel.

Keep the right hip level with the left; there is a tendency to roll that hip up which will change the psoas stretch.

Once you've worked the pose for a few breaths you can try letting the hip roll up if you like. This allows more arch in the back, and a different stretch in the hip that a lot of people like.

You can roll your hip up much further than she is doing in the photo. Although, with the slight roll up of the hip she is getting the maximum psoas stretch Dancers Pose can produce.

For some people rolling the hip way up will create a different psoas stretch. For others the psoas won't stretch with the hip really high.

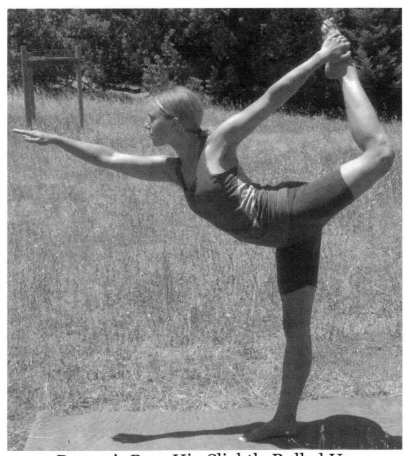

Dancer's Pose Hip Slightly Rolled Up

Standing Lunge Bending

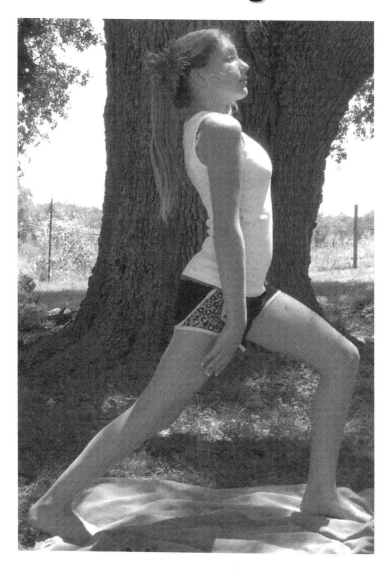

This is another lunge type pose that gives a great stretch for the psoas. It also one of the best Achilles tendon stretches there is.

Start with your left foot forward, right foot back. Bend your right leg so the back heel comes up off the floor. Keep your torso tall with a slight lower back arch.

Keeping your front knee right over the ankle, or at least not past the toes, find a comfortable lunge length that is long, but not too long. It's not a problem if your stance starts too long because you can adjust later when the pose changes.

Press your right heel back. This is a great pose to help your brain learn which way is back by taking your right heel forward then back again to make sure you actually press the heel back.

Notice the stretch in the Achilles tendon and calf. Press your back heel away enough to get a little stretch in those areas. There may even be a little stretch in the posas.

To really stretch the psoas, bend your right leg so the knee goes down fairly far. You may need to shorten your stance to find a comfortable position. Even if your stance is a little shorter than shown in the photo you will get a good psoas stretch.

Keep pressing the heel back to get the best Achilles tendon stretch. Squatting down on the back leg so your weight presses the heel toward the floor will give the ideal Achilles stretch. But, you need to keep your back knee bent enough so the heel is off the floor.

Keep a good back arch throughout for the psoas stretch. Slightly flattening your lower back will increase that stretch.

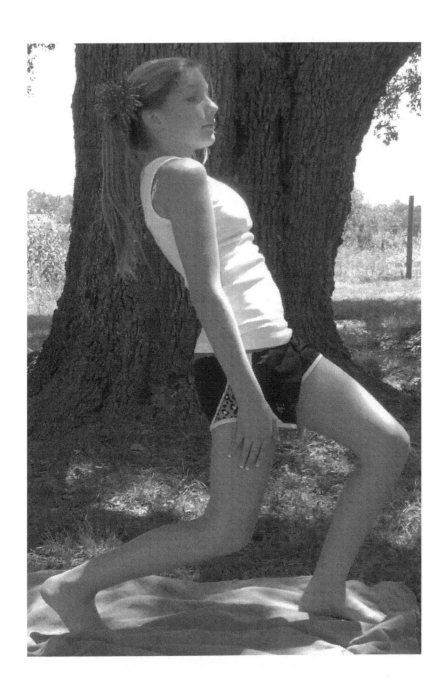

Pigeon Pose

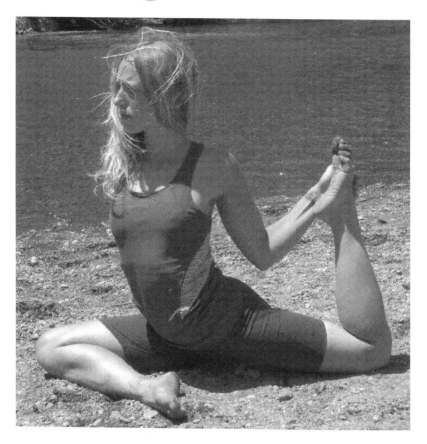

This is an incredible stretch for the hip area, one of the best. The full pose does a great job of stretching the psoas.

Start out in a lunge with your right foot forward and left knee down behind you. Place your right leg down in front of you diagonally at about a 45 degree angle with your knee pointing to the right corner.

There's a tendency to put the leg down so the right knee is pointing forward. If your knee ends up in front of you, shift it over to the right so the leg is at an angle. You'll likely start to feel a stretch in the lower or front hip area with correct positioning.

Place the right foot so the heel is in front of the pubic bone. Closer in is easier, further forward gives a better hip stretch for the more flexible.

Keep your upper body pressed up for the psoas stretch. The higher you press your body up, the more the psoas associated with the back leg will stretch. It also helps to activate the back leg reaching it long behind you.

You can use your hands to press yourself up for more of a backbend. This will help the psoas stretch.

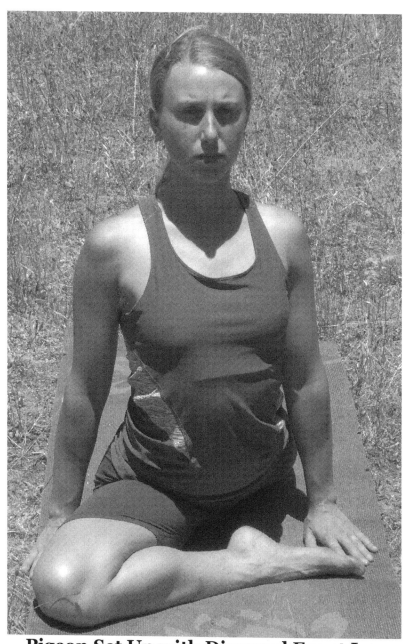

Pigeon Set Up with Diagonal Front Leg

You can get a great quadriceps (front of the thigh) stretch by reaching back and taking your left foot up and forward. Move slowly and pay attention to the front of your thigh because this stretch comes on very quickly. This is the full Pigeon Pose shown in the first photo.

Avoid holding your back leg up without grasping your foot with your hand for too long. Holding the leg up in this position with leg strength alone often causes a cramp in the hamstring.

Relax into the pose allowing your hips to release down for the best hip stretch. You can support your upper body in whatever way is comfortable for you to stretch the front hip area.

Release the back foot and let your upper body down to get an even stronger hip stretch. You can place your elbows on the ground in front of you, or let your body completely down for a stronger stretch. Place your hands in front with your head resting on them if you go all the way down.

Some people are very flexible in the hips. Taking your front foot further forward will increase the hip stretch.

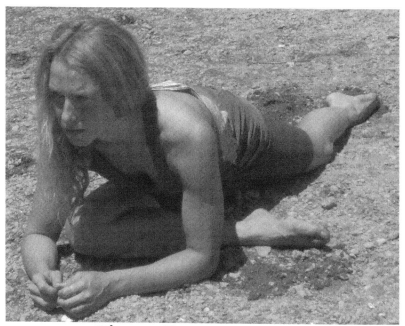

Pigeon Part Way Down

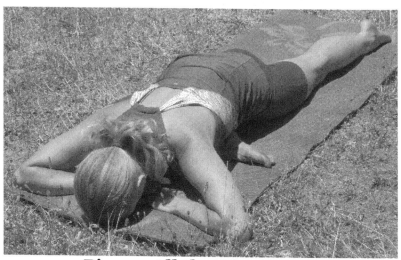

Pigeon All the Way Down

Half Wheel

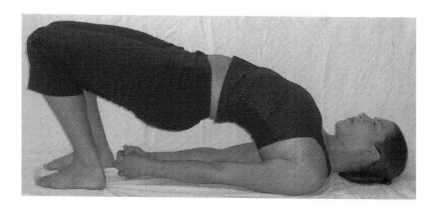

This is a really great psoas stretch for anyone with deep back bend ability. The unsupported version can stretch it, but the supported variation will usually give it a better stretch. It all depends on how tight your psoas is.

Start by lying on your back with your feet on the floor about hip width apart, heels as close to your hips as you comfortably can. Start by first tilting your pelvis as you inhale.

The pelvic tilt is done by simply flattening your lower back into the floor. You can practice that a few times if you are not familiar with the movement. The pelvic tilt alone can feel really good in the lower back and hip areas.

Once the pelvis is tilted, continue inhaling as you lift your hips by pressing your feet into the floor.

Activate your muscles to move your knees away from you as you lift up into the pose. This will help to keep your back safe, and make the lower back more open and the pose solid.

Come deeper into the pose by interlacing your fingers under your back and reaching them toward your feet. As you reach, shift your weight slightly from shoulder to shoulder so your shoulders are pulled further under your back. This will give you more lift and help you to come fully into half wheel.

The supported version is done by taking your hands to your lower back and upper hip area. Once your hands are in a comfortable position let your weight rest into your hands, usually on the heel of the palms.

Or, you can use a foam block in its highest position in the center of your lower back/sacrum area to rest on. Turn the block so the length of the block runs the length of your back. You can bring the block to a lower position if your have less of an arch in your back bend.

Relax into the supported half wheel letting your arms or the block hold all your weight. You can greatly intensify the stretch by walking your feet away from you until your legs are straight, ideally resting on the backs of the heels with the toes pointing up.

With the legs extended is a very deep stretch and should be avoided if you have any back issues, or if there is pain.

Whichever version you do, relax into the stretch letting your belly drop down.

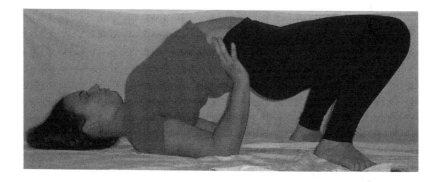

Reclining Thunderbolt

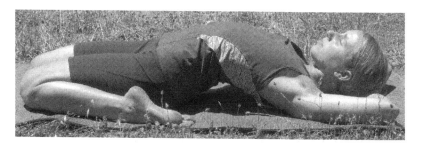

This is another great pose for the psoas which also affects the front thighs. It's another great back arch that can be easily regulated.

Start by sitting between your heels leaning back on your arms behind you. Gently let your upper body down as far as is comfortable for you.

Often, the leg muscles will bunch up. You can change that by rolling your calf muscles outward as you come into sitting on your heels.

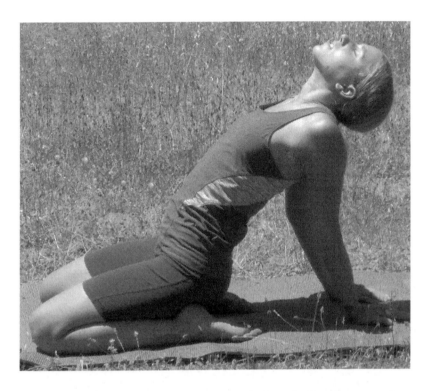

To go deeper, walk your hands back further and rest on your elbows.

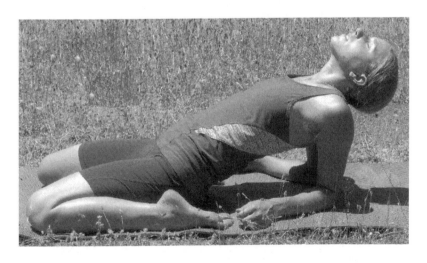

The deepest version is to let your upper body all the way down to the floor like in the first photo. Cross your arms behind your head palms under your shoulders. Rest on your arms making them like a pillow.

Reaching your arms overhead is a nice variation that works the upper body in a different way. Find the one you like best and relax in the pose for a few breaths.

If sitting on your heels causes pain in your knees you can sit on a folded blanket. Avoid using too much height because that can reduce the psoas stretch.

Note: Keeping your knees together throughout is ideal. However, letting them move apart is okay, and you will still get you a great psoas stretch.

Bow Pose

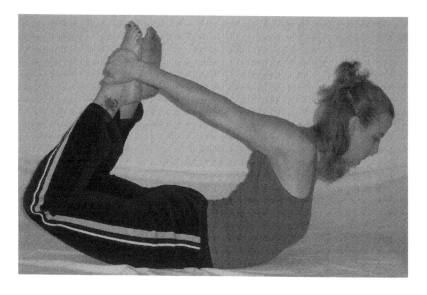

This is another back bend that is good for stretching the psoas. The variation gives it an even better stretch

Start by lying face down. Reach back and take hold of your ankles or feet. Holding the feet is easier if your back bend isn't deep. With an exhale use your leg strength to pull you up into the pose.

Look forward in the pose to arch through the entire spine. Or drop your head slightly if your neck has any discomfort in it.

There is a great variation that allows you to work one side at a time. This is done by doing the pose on your side. This also facilitates working the psoas much deeper than can usually be done in Bow Pose.

The technique is to roll on your side while in Bow Pose. The upper side can be worked more strongly by activating that legs muscles to press the leg more strongly into your hand.

Allow the leg to lift a little further away from your body as the back bend increases on that side. Avoid letting the leg move too far away though because the psoas stretch can decrease with too much distance. Instead, you can pull the leg back down with your arm strength.

Continue to press your foot into your hand. Let your arm and shoulder be pulled back for a nice stretch in that area.

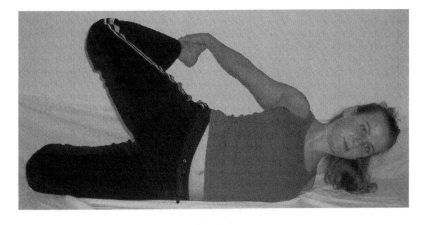

Working the back bend on one side like this can cause a twist in the back. Be careful of this as a twisting arch can cause injury.

Instead of rolling onto your side you might find it easier to lie on your side first, and then take hold of your feet or ankles. Once you are on your side take up a symmetrical side lying Bow Pose, then work the upper leg more as above.

Serpent Pose

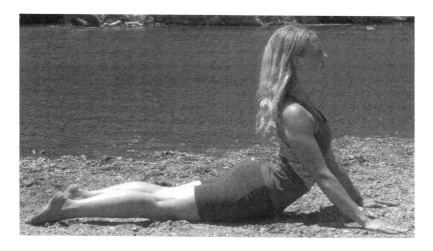

This is a great pose for stretching the back. The psoas is stretched when a subtle adjustment is applied.

There are several variations of Serpent Pose, take time to breath into each one as you progress through the series. The straight arm version is the best for the psoas.

Start by lying down with your legs together or slightly separated, toes pointed. Place your palms on the floor under your shoulders. Let your chin rest on the floor.

The first of the variations is done by taking a breath, and as you exhale lift your upper body.

Only lift with your back strength. Avoid using your arm strength to help you into the pose. Instead, allow your arms and shoulders relax with only their weight resting on the floor. Exhale to come down.

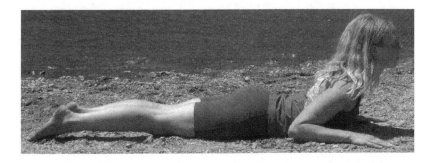

The second variation is to use your arms to press your body up, but only so far as your pubic bone stays on the floor. Exhale as you press yourself up into the pose.

Keep your elbows in alongside your body as you breathe in the pose. Keep your shoulders down and drawing back. Exhale out of the pose.

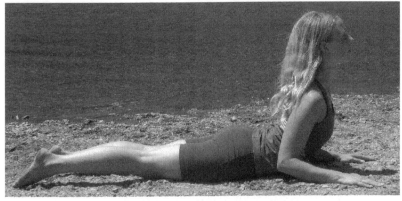

The third variation is to press yourself up as far as you can with straight arms (the first photo above). Exhale as you lift. Continue to lift up out of your shoulders rather than letting your body drop so the shoulders are near your ears.

Use your hands on the floor to gently pull yourself forward to intensify the psoas stretch. Only pull forward enough to lengthen your body, not to slide forward. Ideally, there would be a slight pull on the fronts of the thighs. Exhale when you come down.

The fourth version is to simply rest on your elbows which are placed under your shoulders, forearms forward. Keep your body active so the shoulders aren't hunched up toward your head. Draw your body forward slightly with the arms on the floor for the best psoas stretch.

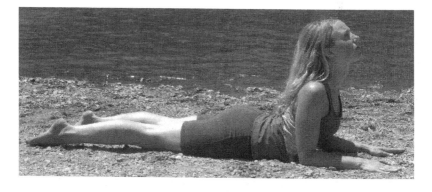

A final variation that people with a flexible back arch will like is to reach your feet toward your head as you reach your head back toward the feet. This can be done with any of the variations, though the Straight Arm Serpent and the Elbow Serpent are the best, especially for the psoas.

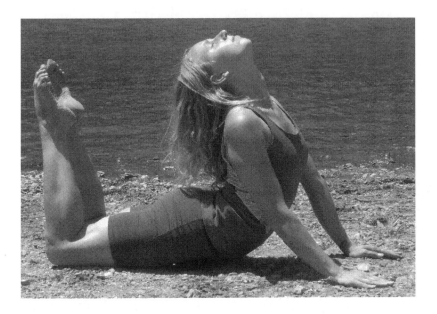

Sitting Arch Twist

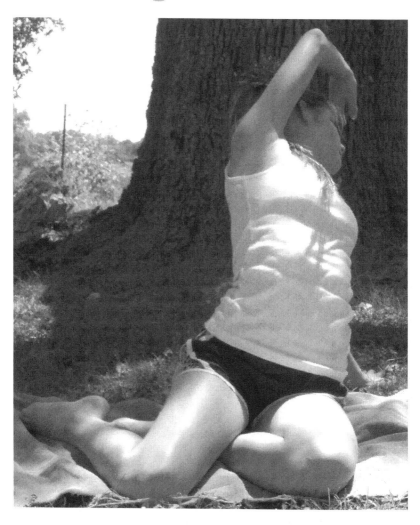

This is a great twist that works strongly into the psoas. It is also one of the best spinal twists there is, and very popular in my classes.

Start by sitting on your feet, then shift your hips to the left so you're sitting to the side of your feet; your feet will be to your right. Twist to the left using your left hand on the floor a foot or more behind you for support.

Use your right hand on your left knee or thigh to help you pull into the twist. Inhale tall, and exhale into the twist.

Next, take your right arm up overhead reaching through your arm to pull you into the twist. The lower back will arch slightly in this position giving you a great arching twist. Avoid working too hard into this if there is any pain at all.

You can go deeper by letting your upper body down. Do this by moving your left hand further away from you so you are leaning further back. Even better is to bend your arm so you are resting on your left elbow

Continue to reach through your upper arm to help you deeper into the twist. Experiment with moving that arm higher or more in front of you to find your best twist and stretch.

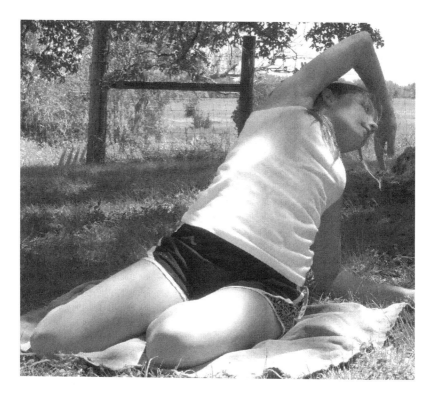

Try to keep your right leg from pulling around with the twist. In fact, move that leg further back if you can for the best right side psoas stretch.

Try releasing the pose enough so you can use your hand to draw the right leg further back, and then go back to the twist. You don't usually need to move the leg far too greatly increase the stretch.

Remember to activate to decrease the arch in your lower back for the best psoas stretch. You may find that there are two positions you like, one for the psoas with less arch, the other with more arch for more stretch in the back.

It is common for the brain to get confused when doing twists. The very common manifestation in this pose is to twist toward the legs rather than away. The reverse direction is actually a good twist, but make sure you are twisting away from your feet for the psoas stretch.

Psoas Self Assist Stretch

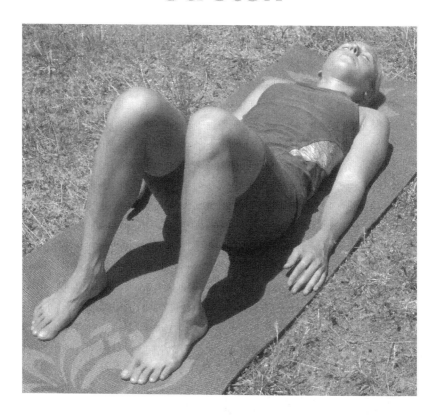

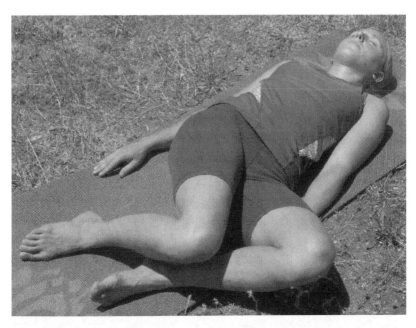

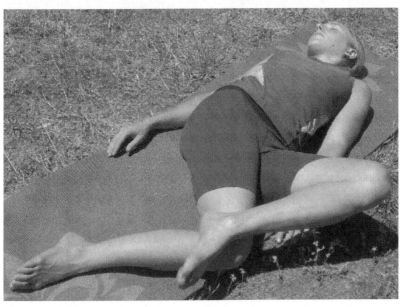

126

This great psoas stretch is very easy to make stronger, or it can be kept gentle as needed. The only issue with this pose is that it can put stress on the knee and hip. Pay attention to these areas to make sure you don't overdo it.

Start by lying on your back with your feet on the floor one to one and a half feet away from your hips. The taller you are the further away they need to be. Have your feet about one and a half hip width apart.

To stretch the right psoas, drop both knees over to the left. Leaving the right leg in place use your left foot to press your right knee down toward the floor. Allow your right foot to roll over as far as it needs to allow the knee to move down.

Try moving your right foot closer or further away from your hips to find the best stretch for you.

Corps Pose

Relaxing after practicing yoga poses is a good way to integrate the work you've been doing. It also gives the energy a chance to flow freely through your body for integration before continuing with your daily activities, or before sleep. And, it can be very purifying for the body and thoughts.

Start by lying comfortably on your back with your legs extended and spread fairly wide. Have them at least wide enough so the feet fall over to the sides on their own when relaxed.

If your lower back is tight you can put something soft under your knees to relieve the pressure. Or, position a chair so you can rest your lower legs and feet on the seat to completely relieve any lower back pressure.

Have your arms to the sides, palms up. If the palms are down, we naturally tend to press the floor which isn't conducive to relaxing. Have the arms a foot or more away from your body.

Take a few diaphragmatic breaths; breathing so your belly rises and falls with the chest not moving at all. This breath stimulates the part of the nervous system that relaxes the body while chest breathing will make the body tense up. A hand on your chest will let you know when you are successful with diaphragmatic breathing since your chest won't be moving as you breathe.

After a minute or two (or more if you like) of diaphragmatic breathing allow your breath to relax to what is natural for you. More diaphragmatic breathing is fine as it will help you to relax, but only if it is natural.

Then, start consciously relaxing the various parts of your body. Take a few breaths with each part as you focus on relaxing each area.

If there is more tension in a particular body part you can give that area extra relaxation by bringing your attention to the body part that is tense as you inhale a little more deeply, then let go as you release your breathe and the tight area.

Start the relaxation with your feet, then the calves, and on up into the thighs. Allow your hips and buttocks to relax feeling yourself sink into the floor.

Let the relaxation move up into your belly, allowing your abdominals to relax and release down through the torso, and through the organs of the belly. Allow everything to release down and into your lower back as it relaxes.

Then, bring your attention into your chest allowing it to relax and release down into the middle back and then the upper back. Allow the tops of your shoulders to relax and release down.

Let the relaxation out into your shoulders, upper arms, forearms, wrists, and hands. Allow your arms to fully relax and sink into the floor.

Then bring your attention into your face, allowing your face to relax. Let your forehead relax, the scalp and eyes. Allow your eyes to sink deep into their sockets as they relax.

Allow your jaw to relax. Relax your mouth and tongue so that it releases and drops deeper into your mouth.

Let the relaxation drain down through your head and into the back of your head. Feel the back of your head relax as though sinking into the floor.

Take a few minutes to relax, whatever is a comfortable amount of time for you. You can set a timer if you like, preferably one that will turn itself off so you don't have to move quickly.

When you are ready, start coming back slowly by bringing your attention back to yourself, feeling your body and breath as your attention comes back to you lying on the floor.

Start moving your fingers and toes a little.
Gradually let that movement increase into your
hands and your feet, then into your arms and the
legs. Let your breath deepen as you come back.

Once you are back to yourself, roll onto your
right side and relax there for a minute or two.
Then very gently, when you're ready, press
yourself up to sitting to complete the class.

About the Author

Kalidasa is currently based in the Russian River area of Northern California. He is a long time yoga instructor, holistic healer and tantra practitioner. He has worked with individuals and groups for over 35 years.

His strong desire to help people learn to help themselves has led him to writing books on health, yoga and tantric techniques. His current books are listed below.

He has spent his life meditating, teaching yoga and developing unique techniques that that have impacted thousands of people. He has recently come out of seclusion to offer even more information for the benefit of others.

He is the developer of Self Adjusting Technique (SAT), a method of doing gentle adjustments on yourself so chiropractic adjustments can be avoided.

The simple adjustments don't require force or cracking, so they are much more appealing to people who don't like that type of work. You can learn about SAT and other healing techniques as well as what his healing private sessions are by visiting http://selfadjustingtechnique.com

His new site, http://kalidasa.com has more information about Kalidasa and some of the practices mentioned in this book. http://yogawithkalidasa.com is his yoga site.

You can contact him through his sites about private or group sessions.

Other Books by Kalidasa Brown

Self Adjusting Technique

This book teaches you how to do adjustments on yourself so you can avoid visits to the chiropractor. The adjustments are very gentle with no force or cracking involved.

The adjustments are based on the principle that your body goes in and out of alignment all the time. The body simply adjusts itself by means of muscles pulling on the bones combined with movement to easily slip joints back into proper alignment.

Tight muscles prevent this natural realignment, but you can do the same thing with gentle pressure and easy movements to realign yourself naturally.

Included are adjustment techniques for the neck, back, hips and ribs.

Adrenal Fatigue: Get Your Life Back

Adrenal fatigue is the hidden condition that most doctors know little to nothing about. Multiple symptoms and conditions completely baffle most doctors who just throw medications at the problems to see what might help. Now you can truly take your life back by understanding this little known but all too common condition.

Eliminate Fat Hormones for Weight Loss and Health -Lose Weight and Prevent Cancer with Supplements

Estrogenic cancer is the most deadly type of cancer. It is caused by the liver not making the hormone water solvable for elimination. Estrogen is also the hormone that makes fat deposit in the body. Giving the liver the nutrients needed to eliminate estrogen both prevents cancer, and aids in weight loss.

Yoga for Lower Back Pain

This is an easy to follow yoga class with poses that are of great help to most back pain issues. Plenty of information on how to care for your back is included.

Tantra for the Up and Not Coming Man, And the Woman that Wants to Help Him Keep Going All Night

This book contains practical Tantra Yoga for men and women who want sex to last far beyond the average 10 or 15 minutes. It includes simple exercises that will help men gain the ability to restrain ejaculation so sex can continue indefinitely.

It also contains a yoga class to increase his abilities to an extremely advanced level. The class also increases energy for women and men. That can increase the length of time for lovers to spend together.

While this book is written for men, women can learn how to support their partner for both to experience more pleasure and intimacy together.

Floor Yoga Class

A simple yet complete yoga class that is done completely on the floor. Perfect for the beginner or limited yoga practitioner.

Made in the USA
San Bernardino, CA
21 June 2018